A Dietary Connection for POTS, EDS and MCAS

by

Lynne D M Noble

Independently published 2020

About the Author

Lynne Noble was born in 1953 in Huddersfield, West Yorkshire. From a very early age, Lynne showed an interest in nutrition and genetics avidly reading any books that she could get her hands on at the time.

Initially, Lynne studied orthopaedics but events led her to work with the elderly mentally infirm. Here, her interest in neurodegenerative disorders and pain syndromes developed.

Lynne undertook rigorous programmes of study, completing her Cert Ed., (FE) BSc (Hons) and Adv. Dip Education simultaneously before moving onto her M.Ed.

From there she took further demanding programmes in Human Nutrition, Pharmacology, Neuroscience, Genetics and Immunology. During this time, she was given many prestigious awards for her academic work. It was noted then that Lynne was not afraid of tackling difficult subjects.

She began her law degree but ill health prevented her from pursuing this. However, in this time, she moved from being a foster parent to adoptive parent.

She has been instrumental in setting up projects in the community for disadvantaged groups.

She is a member of the Guild of Health Writers and the British Union of Journalists.

Now retired, she lives with her husband in a historic Georgian riverside town in the West Midlands. She enjoys gardening, watching her husband bowling and researching.

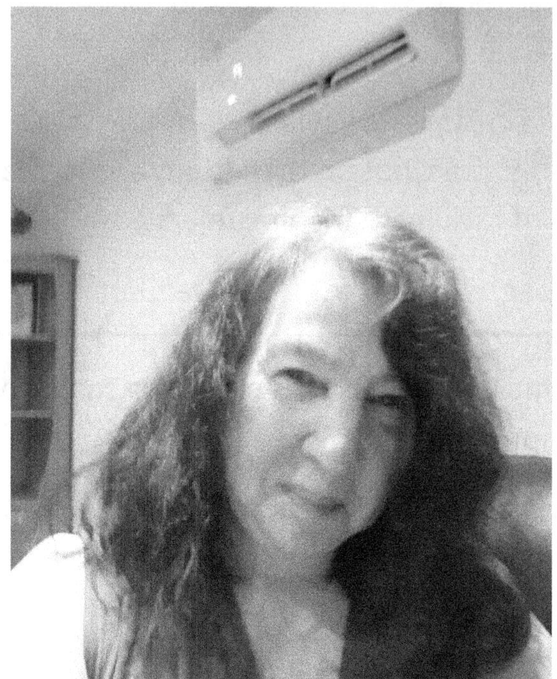

Author Lynne Noble –aged 67 years - at home

https://quintessentiallylynne.weebly.com/nutritional-medicine.html

Preface

I became personally acquainted with Postural Orthostatic Tachycardia Syndrome (POTS) when I was seventeen. I recall suddenly feeling 'peculiarly' light headed and weak on a short walk down to the shop. I propped myself up against the wall hoping that the moment would pass. It did not and I slid gracefully down the wall and sat there in a semi-conscious state until I felt strong enough to get up again.

I suppose, like many, I put it down to overwork, missing breakfast and stress, among others. None of these applied but you look for the obvious causes when medical knowledge is limited and you have no further answers.

I did have a prolonged bout of whatever virus was going around when I was in the middle of my GCE's. It laid me low for months. When most teenagers were out dancing, I could barely muster enough energy to stay up until 8pm.

I had never heard of the term Chronic Fatigue Syndrome or post viral syndrome then but looking back, I can see that my symptoms would have fitted the bill.

All my problems appeared to stem from that time. I had been an active child but found getting through an ordinary day, difficult. I had permanent brain fog and, of course, I began to have these peculiar bouts of light headedness and weakness sometimes ending in brief unconscious bouts.

Now, we know a great deal more about this disorder and it is not unusual to find that it began shortly after a viral infection. However, it is also linked to many other conditions maybe reflecting its diverse aetiology.

POTS is linked to Ehlers Danlos Syndrome, Chronic Fatigue Syndrome, dysmotility and neurological conditions, to name but a few.

Often the first sign of these conditions, that people actually take notice of is POTS. You can't hardly ignore it when it happens.

In my case I had a connective tissue disorder known as Ehlers Danlos syndrome. I did not know it then. It wasn't identified for years until I was referred to rheumatology after sustaining numerous tendon injuries over prolonged periods.   Even then, I wasn't told of my diagnosis although it is there in my notes. I was given splints in the hope that this would help with my problem and discharged.

The splints did help with my lower limb tendon problems but not the problems with my upper limbs.   They did not help with the chronic fatigue, numerous soft tissue injuries in my back, the headaches, the cervical injuries, the peculiar ability of my jaw to lock or indeed any of the other odd and apparently unrelated symptoms that I had.

Indeed, when I went to a new GP for my initial appointment, she threw up her hands in horror and said, 'Do you actually know how thick your notes are?'

I did find my way to physiotherapy on a number of occasions but the connection between the frequent upper limb injuries and those in my lower limbs did not appear to be understood by those in the health profession.

In the end, as chronic pain often does, it became a part of me. I felt lucky if I could get through one day without being in pain. I assumed it was just one of life's quirks but now and again I did wonder why I had so many joint, muscle and tendon problems when it was clear so many other people didn't.

I did not know then that POTS would be a lifelong companion although, for most part, I have put it to bed.

POTS has been recognised since 1940. It is mostly seen in women of child bearing age although it is found rarely, outside these parameters. It is, for example, found in older groups.

However, we are not looking at a syndrome with one underlying cause. POTS can have a number of causes and some may have a significant and debilitating impact on the individual's life. Thorough investigation is needed before tailored treatment can be administered.

Sometimes the underlying mechanism cannot be ascertained and this can make treatment difficult. However, the underlying causes do appear to differ between younger and older adults with the syndrome.

I have a thirst for life, the spirit of an adventurer and in order to fulfil this side of me, I have had to learn how to master POTS rather than the other way around.

I learned what was likely to trigger it. That was empowering because then, the responsibility of avoiding those triggers was in my hands. I was the one holding the reins, I was the one in control.

This book was written with the intention of exploring POTS – what it is and how it can be addressed with lifestyle changes including better nutrition.

Life is meant to be lived to the full so our mastery of chronic conditions is an essential player in this process.

What is this POTS syndrome?

A syndrome is a collection of signs and symptoms that occur together and signal a particular disorder or condition.

Signs and symptoms have different definitions although they are often used simultaneously. Signs are those events that the medic notices in their examination such as raised blood pressure or a slower than expected heartbeat.

Symptoms are those that the patient tends to report such as pain, brain fog or feeling colder than usual.

 The names of syndromes generally describe the more salient features of this cluster of signs and symptoms although in some cases it may reflect the name of the individual who first recognised that a particular group of signs and symptoms kept occurring.

Thus Postural Orthostatic Tachycardia Syndrome adequately describes the way that the heartbeat increases rapidly when changes in position occur.

Alternatively, syndromes can be named after the person who identified the cluster of symptoms that gave rise to a recognised disorder.

Elhers Danlos Syndrome (EDS) identifies the two medics who gave their name to this connective tissue disorder.

EDS has been around for a long time. It was described by Hippocrates in 400 BC and so could be considered one of the most ancient descriptions of connective tissue disorders.

However, it was not until 1901 that it was described as a specific condition by Edvard Ehlers. Seven years later, in 1908, Henri Danlos proposed that fundamental features of this syndrome were skin extensibility and fragility.

Although the salient features of POTS are the postural change and associated tachycardia, there are many other signs and symptoms which accompany this syndrome which include:

- Heart palpitations
- Light-headedness or fatigue
- Weakness and sweating and internal tremors
- Fainting also known as syncope
- Brain fog – inability to concentrate, think, recall
- Poor sleep patterns
- Nausea
- Headaches
- Irritable bowels syndrome type symptoms
- Shortness of breath

In my case, it would often start if I got too hot. Sometimes I would feel faint very shortly after I had eaten something or even during a casual walk down to the shops.

 I don't normally eat crisps but I found that if I took some with me and ate them, if I felt faint, then it stopped the process from progressing.

Another trigger for me was the antibiotic, clarithromycin which I was prescribed when I had a bout of community pneumonia. A condition known as Mast Cell Activation Syndrome (MCAS) and often associated with POTS appeared to be at play here.

I had only just moved to my new home and did not have my usual apothecary set up. It was in one of the many boxes lying about the place and I could not remember which one.

 Nevertheless, I had an initial appointment with my new GP who diagnosed pneumonia. I was prescribed clarithromycin which the bacterial pneumonia responded well to, apparently.

The GP was surprised that I could still be walking around and asked me to obtain and start the course of antibiotics as soon as possible.

On the way back home from the chemist, I purchased a takeaway coffee and took the first capsule. I stopped and chatted to some friends for a while then set off home again. I felt peculiarly light-headed and my heart felt as though it was pounding.

I put it down to the infection and reached home without problem. Whatever had occurred had ended. It had been a temporary and minor aberration.

At 7pm, I took the second capsule. A friend called some minutes later and I recall that I could not take in what she was say and wished that she would go so that I could go and lie down.

I eventually stumbled to the settee. As luck would have it, I had begun to sort my medical gadgets out and my oximeter was on a tray. I barely had strength to use it but it showed that my heart rate was over 150 bpm.

 My husband rang emergency. Two paramedics turned up and I was despatched to the crash room at our local hospital where my pulse dipped and rose in random fashion before settling after a couple of hours.

That was the last time that I took clarithromycin but it appeared that a dysautonomia and allergic response were at play here.

The percentage overlap between MCAS and POTS is not known even though there is a known association. This is partially down to the fact that both conditions are poorly understood anyway.

Mast cells are associated with allergies. Those with hay fever, asthma, urticaria and angieoedema will be well acquainted with mast cells. They secrete many substances which are involved in the inflammatory response such as histamine. Histamine causes swelling, redness and histamine.

'Nettle rash' - which most children will be familiar with – occurs as a response of mast cells to the chemicals that flow through the fine needle like hairs found on the stems and leaves. When faced with a toxic substance, mast cells release histamine which coordinates a response to the invading substance.

Other common contenders for activating mast cells are peanuts, cat dander and bee stings.

When mast cells are activated on a regular basis and repeatedly produces   recognised signs and symptoms then it is labelled Mast Cell Activation Syndrome.

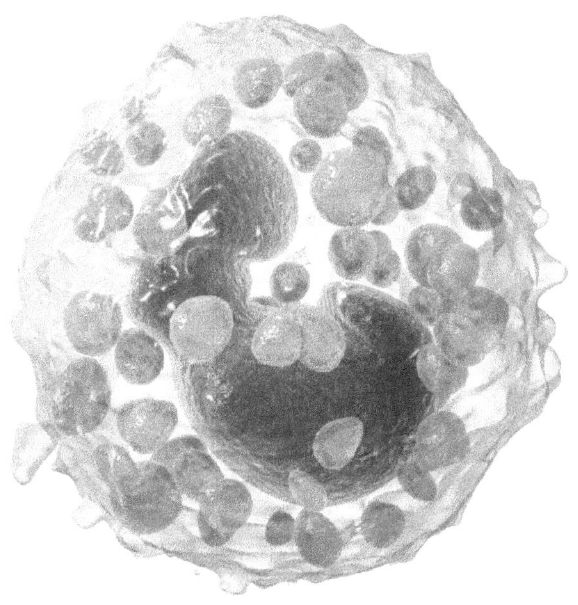

Mast cells release histamine when activated

Some of the signs and symptoms found in MCAS are also to be found in POTS.   MCAS include:

- Abdominal pain
- Light-headedness
- Brain fog and memory difficulties
- Itching, wheezing and other allergy type reactions

It may be that there is a subset of individuals whose POTS may be caused by an abnormally high number of mast cells. Alternatively, something may be causing the mast cells to be activated too easily.

Angieoedema is a swelling of the deeper layers of skin tissue. The swelling is due to activated mast cells. You will find it angieoedema as part of a severe allergic reaction known as anaphylaxis which can be life-threatening. However, it is also found in a condition known as mastocytosis where there appears to be an excessive amount of mast cells as opposed to a greater susceptibility to be activated.

There is also a condition called idiopathic angieoedema. It is not fuelled by an IgE reaction but nevertheless, causes similar symptoms.

Idiopathic angieoedema refers to a cause that is not known. There can be physical causes such as heat and pressure which contribute to the swelling rather than different proteins such as those found in nuts.

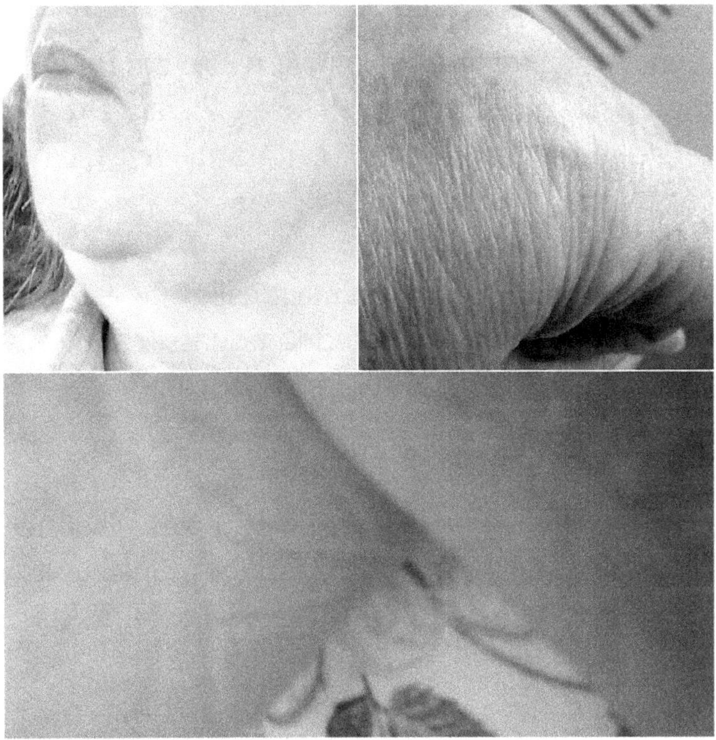

Top left: angieoedema swelling beginning in throat area

Top right: urticarial rash

Bottom picture: demographics (skin writing) due to fluid

Although the presence of allergic conditions points to a diagnosis of MCAS related POTS, there is a blood test that looks for an enzyme called tryptase which can provide further confirmation.

Tryptase is derived from mast calls and is found in greater than expected amounts especially after an anaphylactic type episodes.

 The presence of elevated levels of this enzyme may be a relief because this provides evidence that mast cells are the ones responsible for symptoms and treatments are available for this.

 Levels of tryptase   can be measured by collecting a 24- hour urine sample. Nevertheless, the tryptase level may be found to be normal. In that case, MCAS would not be responsible for POTS.

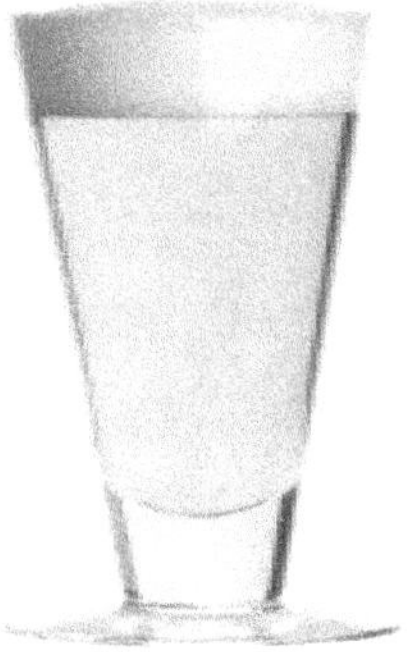

A 24 hour-urine sample may be used to measure tryptase levels which are elevated in MCAS

Symptoms caused by mast cells are due to their contents being released so that these chemicals can respond to injury or infection.

These substances include:

- Histamine
- Leukotrienes
- prostaglandins

Leukotrienes are biologically active compound which originally derived from white blood cells. They are the metabolites of arachidonic acid and are inflammatory in nature.

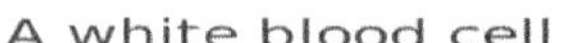

A white blood cell

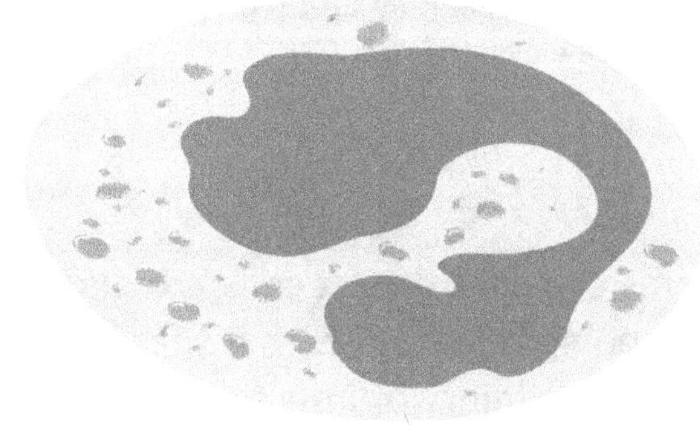

Leukotrienes originated from white blood cells

A metabolite is just the end product of a process. They can be used by the body to effect an action.

Leukotrienes are a major player in allergy types symptoms. They are well known for their negative effects on asthma and help to constrict airways.

In addition, they increase the permeability of tiny blood vessels causing leakiness and swelling of the tissues. The constriction and swelling in the airways can make breathing much harder.

Arachidonic acid can be converted to pro inflammatory substances or anti-inflammatory ones. You can be sure that if you suffer from asthma or other allergies that arachidonic acid has been converted to an inflammatory substance.

However, this conversion cannot take place if there aren't many spare electrons to disrupt the cell wall membranes. These membranes are largely composed of fats which oxidise easily. Therefore, a diet high in fresh fruit and vegetables foods are essential to prevent this happening.

However, trace elements like selenium and zinc have antioxidant capacity and prevent cellular damage.

Arachidonic acid is found in the omega 6 polyunsaturated fatty acids. Sunflower oil is a popular source. It appears to be added to most readymade foods including biscuits, cakes and ready meals. It is ubiquitous and can impact negatively on health when not balanced appropriately with the omega 3 fatty acids.

Margarines are generally made from sunflower oil although there are some margarines which contain monounsaturated oils like olive oil.

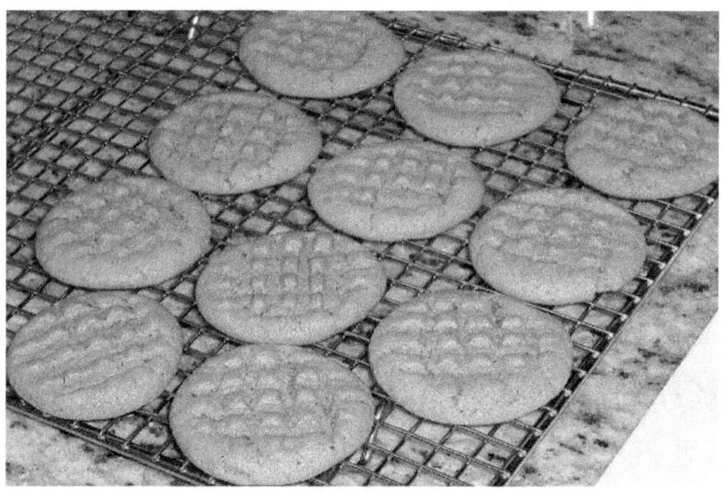

Biscuits made with margarine from sunflower oil contain high amounts of inflammatory omega 6.

our consumption of PUFA's has risen dramatically since their introduction. They have now replaced the more stable saturated fats such as lard, dripping and butter that were the mainstay of the UK diet until around the early 1970's when the apparently 'healthy' benefits of omega polyunsaturated fatty acids were heavily marketed.

The return to more natural fats would be beneficial in cases of MCAS induced POTS. Saturated fats are stable fats and do not give rise to inflammation nor do they activate mast cells.

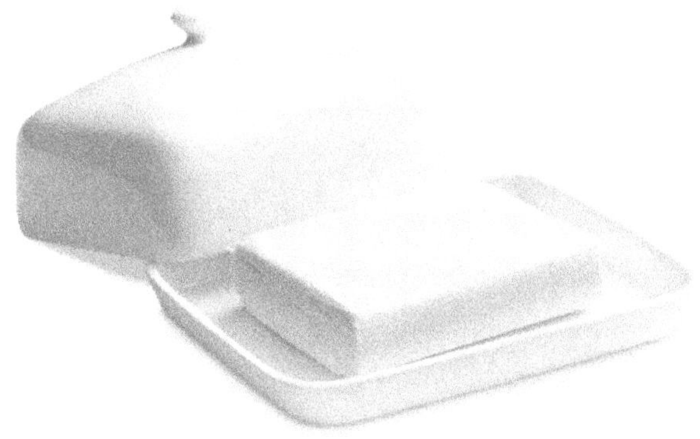

Butter is a stable fat and less likely to activate mast cells than the inflammatory omega 6 oils

Contrary to belief, they do not raise cholesterol levels. They provide reasonable amounts of vitamin D. individuals who eat saturated fats tend to have healthy unwrinkled skin. Those whose main form of fatty acids are the omega 6 fatty acids tend to have unhealthy looking skin that forms lines easily.

Most people are familiar with the concept of eating 'five a day.' That is, eating a wide variety of fresh vegetables and fruit with a diversity of colours and antioxidants oozing out of them. A diet like this can often prevent the conversion of arachidonic acid to pro inflammatory substances especially if they are not overly cooked.

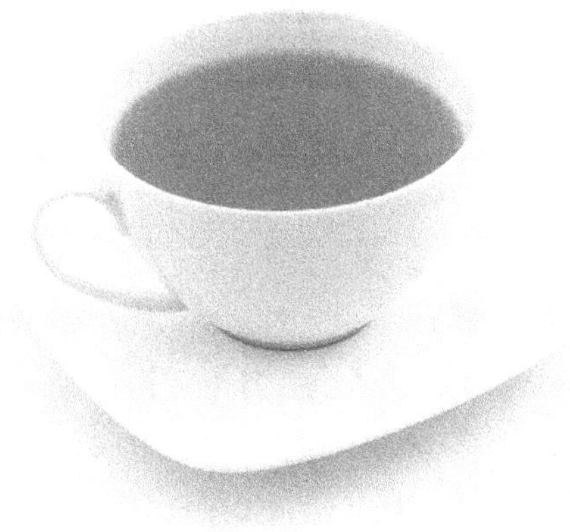

A cup of tea contains quercetin

The main antioxidant with particular benefits for MCAS is quercetin.

Quercetin is particularly bountiful in onions, apples, tea and coffee. All of these had been a daily part of my diet for as long as I remember. I am sure that this is one of the reasons that I do not tend to suffer from the common inflammatory disorders as many of my contemporaries do.

Nevertheless, one day, after suffering some facial swelling for a number of weeks, I supplemented with 500mg of quercetin. This is a considerably larger amount than I would be able to obtain from my normal diet.

The following day all the subtle swelling around my nose and eyes had gone. I looked a totally different person – younger and brighter – without the puffiness that accompanies allergic reactions, however mild.

Quercetin has been the best dietary supplement for my underlying vulnerability to MACS. I now take 500mg daily and find it far better than any antihistamine. All this and without the negative side effects than accompany antihistamines.

Of course quercetin may not be the best supplement for everyone. Genetics play their part in deciding what is most suitable for any individual.

Preventing the conversion of leukotrienes from the parent arachidonic acid can be achieved by blocking an enzyme called lipoxygenase.

There are a number of food sources which can inhibit this process, one of which just happens to be quercetin.

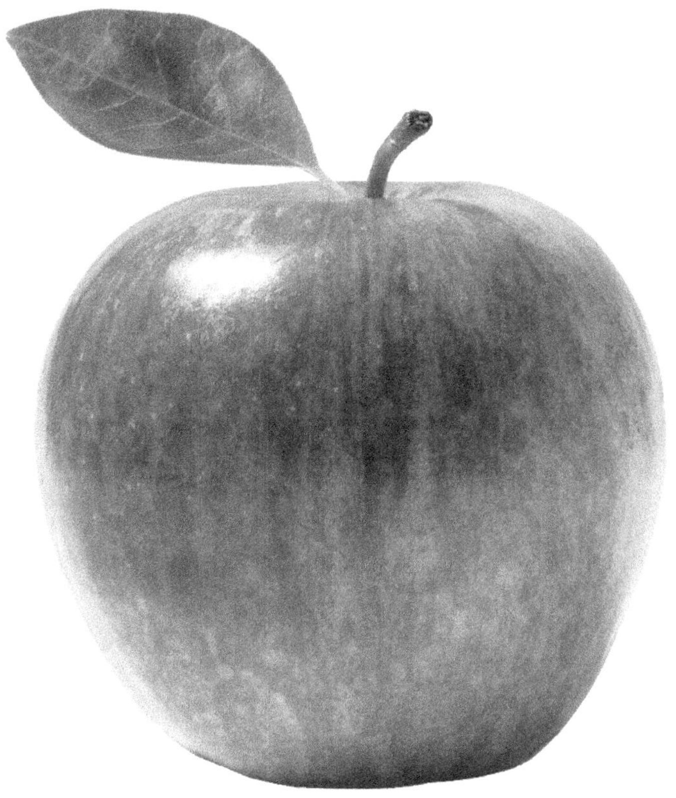

Apples are good sources of quercetin

Curcumin is a good inhibitor of lipoxygenase but the monoeic fatty acids are perhaps most useful inhibitors for day to day use.

Monoenoic fatty acids

A number of long chain monoenoic fatty acids were found to have an effect on lipoxygenase (5-LO) activity.

Studies show that oleic acid, found in olive oil, has by far the greatest inhibitory effect on 5-LO. Oleic acid is a monounsaturated fatty acid that is found in goodly amounts in olive oil and macadamia nuts.

If you can get into the habit of pouring 10 mls or so over a meal, or into soup, it can make difference as to whether MCAS manifests itself.

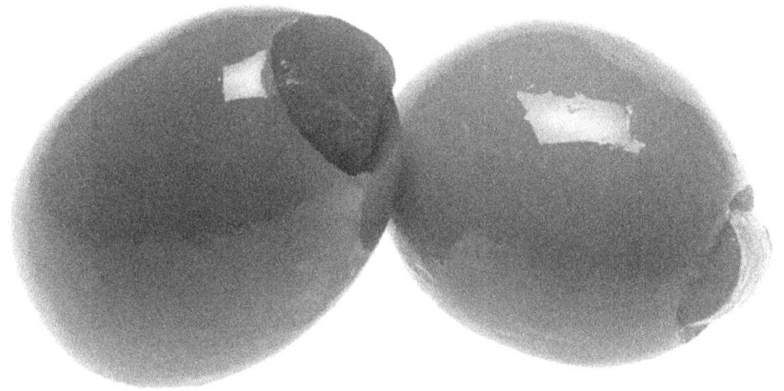

Olives are full of monoeic acid

Histamine and Prostaglandins

When we encounter painful stimuli, chemicals called prostaglandins, from mast cells, are released alongside the stimulus. They increase the sensitivity of pain receptors. This has some value in that we are immediately likely to retract from something that could injure us as well as 'guard' the injured area which would aid healing.

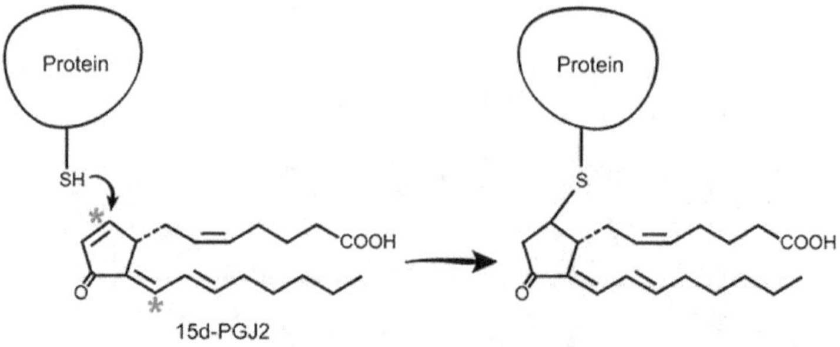

Prostaglandins are chemical substances that can promote pain.

Prostaglandins can either promote or reduce inflammation depending on nutritional intake at the time.

 Fish oils contain high concentrations of omega-3 fatty acids. These have been proven to shift the balance from the prostaglandins that increase inflammation to those that lessen it.

The best source of omega 3 fatty acids is oily fish such as mackerel, salmon and fresh tuna. Tinned tuna does not contain omega 3 fatty acids, so while tuna may be a good source of protein it will not contribute to your omega 3 fatty acid needs.

Ginger is also beneficial for counteracting symptoms related to prostaglandin release. My cousin says that it has been the only treatment that has worked on the pain of an arthritic knee.

Histamine is a vasoactive amine which has an important role in the early acute inflammatory response after infection or injury. (An amine is just a substance that is derived from ammonia).

Histamine is stored in the granules of mast cells, basophils and platelets.

Histamine is released from cells by stimuli which include acute inflammation caused by injury or infection.

Histamine increases vasodilation - that is it widens blood vessels. It also makes them more permeable too and this allows the entry of immune system cells to the site of injury or infection so that it can be dealt with effectively.

Histamine is the main chemical mediator and directs immune system substances to the site of injury. This may include cells to specifically deal with infection or cells required for the repair to any injury to tissue. This coordinated process inevitably causes swelling. Swelling presses on sensitive nerve endings causing pain. Limiting movement, due to pain, can be beneficial and aid healing.

If histamine release appears to be a particular problem in MCAS then quercetin should be tried first.

The recommended amount is 500mg although in severe cases of histamine release, 1000mg in divided doses may be taken. However, it is always better to take advice from a qualified nutritionist if you are considering this.

At this point it is probably a good time to round up what we have learned so far.

- POTS has a number of symptoms in common with MCAS
- An enzyme – tryptase – is elevated in those whose POTS is likely to be due to mast cell activation

- The contents of mast cells produce allergy type symptoms such as those found in hay fever and asthma. Wheezing, itching, tearing of the eyes and swelling are common.
- There are a number of types of chemicals that are released from mast cells. These include histamines, leukotrienes and prostaglandins.
- Quercetin – at 500mg supplementation – tends to work very well for allergic symptoms, although there are other dietary supplements that can help
- Saturated fats are not inflammatory in nature like the omega 6 poly unsaturated fatty acids. In addition, the omega 3 fatty acids can ameliorate the effect of degranulation of mast cells.
- If the tryptase levels are not raised and there has been a diagnosis of POTS, then the underlying cause is highly unlikely to be caused by over enthusiastic mast cells releasing their contents into bodily systems with all the havoc that can cause. If that is the case, then another cause must be looked for.

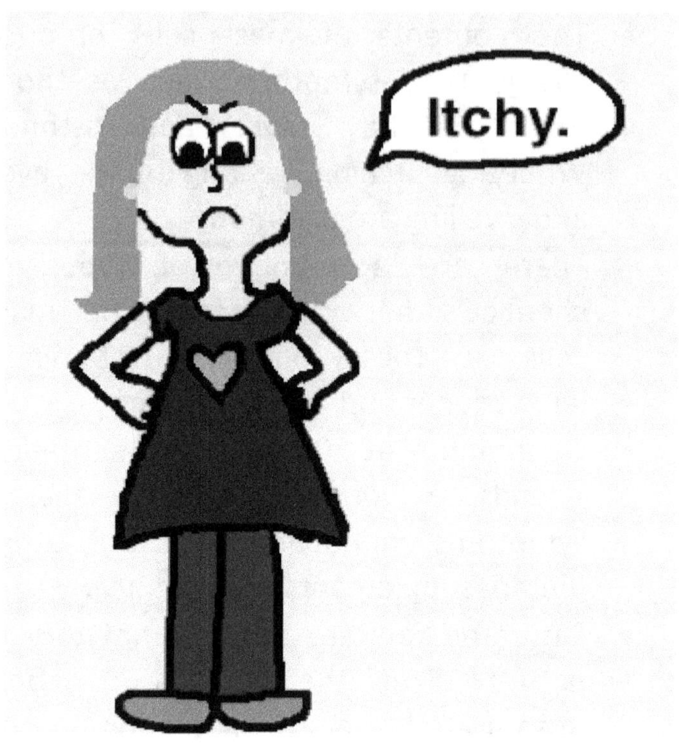

Excessive histamine can make you feel itchy.

Three main substances released from mast cells in MCAS, traditional treatment and potential dietary interventions

substance	Traditional treatment	Dietary supplements or interventions
Prostaglandins	Non-steroidal anti-inflammatory drugs such as ibuprofen and aspirin	Ginger, curcumin and omega three fatty acids especially EPA
leukotrienes	Montelukast	Monoeic fatty acids like olive oil, curcumin, quercetin
histamines	Antihistamines such as Loratidine or the H2 receptors like ranitidine for	Quercetin, bromelain found in pineapple

	nausea and abdominal pain	

Omalizumab – a common prescription drug - blocks binding of Immunoglobulin E to its receptors and, as such can dampen down mast cell reactivity. This can reduce anaphylaxis episodes.

However, many prescription drugs have unwanted side effects and these can be worse than the original condition help was sought for. It makes sense that the main focus of the management of MCAS, and associated POTS, should major on avoiding triggers, reducing stress, keeping to a well-balanced diet high in antioxidants and avoiding over exertion.

Although there is a significant association between POTS and MCAS, the treatment for POTS is different. Here the focus is on keeping the blood pressure raised, by, for example, increasing sodium in the diet. This appears to be the easiest way of responding to POTS.

Compression garments are also recommended as they prevent fluid from pooling in the lower extremities. Nevertheless, they are uncomfortable to wear and can be difficult to put on and take off.

Beta blockers are a third option as they reduce the potential for tachycardia to occur. However, there appear to be a number of side effects associated with prescription medication and people with MCAS appear to be particularly susceptible to medications in general.

Increasing foods which contain the amino acid, tyrosine, can raise blood pressure in a therapeutic manner. We will revisit this subject later.

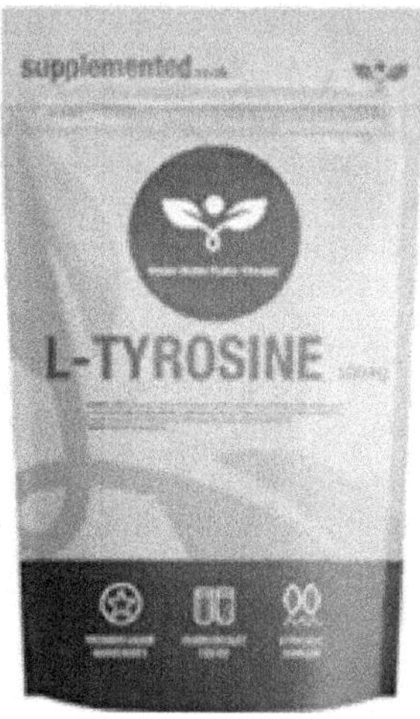

Tyrosine is able to elevate blood pressure and comes in supplemental form. It may be useful for POTS.

Caution has also to be applied when taking diuretics such as Furosemide which is commonly prescribed for those with water retention. They work by making you urinate more.   In doing so they flush sodium, chloride, potassium and water out of your body. These minerals are vitally important for life itself.   When deficiency and imbalance occurs then ill health will be the result.

As fluid is lost, your blood pressure drops. When you are particularly prone to dysautonomia this can increase the threshold for POTS associated syncope to occur.

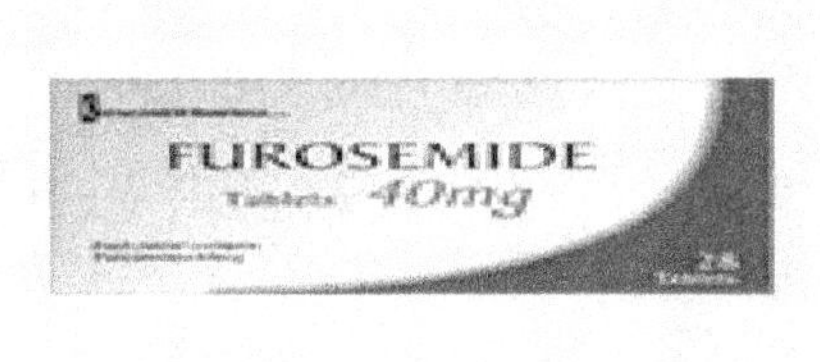

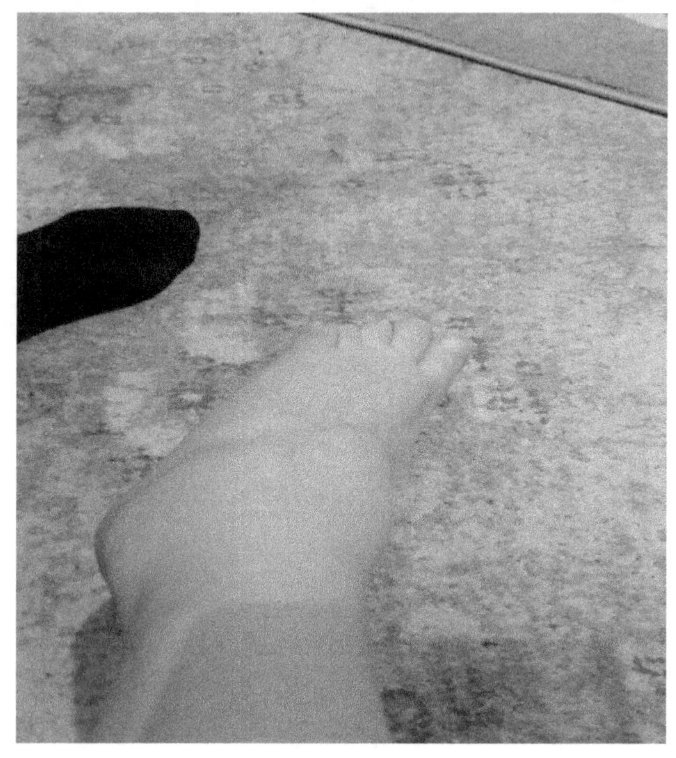

Pooling of fluid in lower limbs is common in POTS and MACS. Diuretics may be given to try and correct this swelling, but it can make you more susceptible to episodes of POTS.

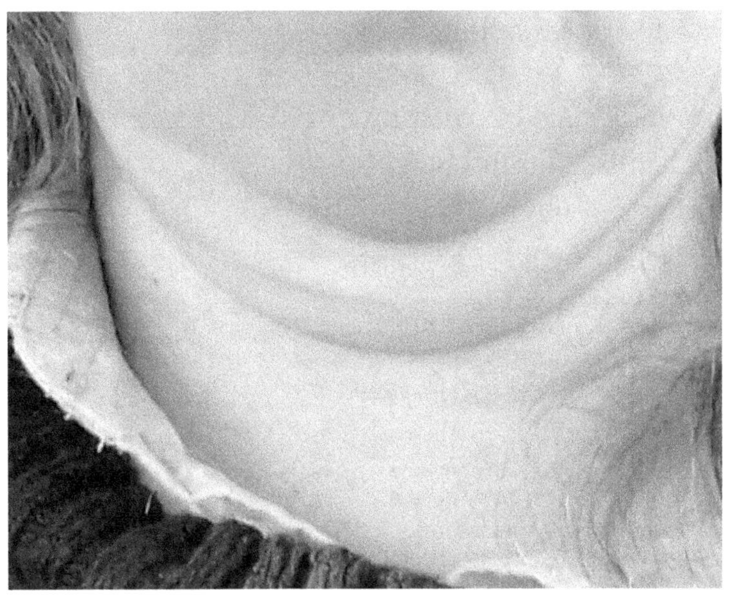

A good example of mast cell activated angieoedema. The patient had an Epipen for such times but has not had to use it since taking supplemental quercetin.

There are a number of other prescription drugs which can worsen POTS. These should be stopped, if possible, to see if it improves POTS.

These medications include:

- Angiotensin converting enzyme inhibitors
- Calcium channel blockers
- Monoamine oxidase inhibitors
- Tricyclic antidepressants
- phenothiazine's

There is some evidence that reducing carbohydrate in the diet may also help POTS. High carbohydrate diets result in lower blood pressure. Conversely, a diet that is higher in protein appeared to raise blood pressure.

The ability of a high protein diet to raise blood pressure may be due to the levels of the amino acid in the food being eaten. Hormones are formed from combinations of amino acids and send messages to target organs directing them to perform some action.

High carbohydrate diets have the ability to raise blood sugar levels quickly but there is a corresponding surge in insulin release. This results in a rapid drop in blood sugar know as reactive hypoglycaemia.   It is often accompanied by symptoms such as:

- shaking
- internal tremors
- weakness
- brain fog
- anxiety
- tachycardia
- sweating
- headaches
- irritability

Reactive hypoglycaemia has a different underlying cause than POTS but is often mistaken for it initially. There is a relationship between diabetes and POTS, too, but we will come to that later.

A diet followed by diabetics will often address the problem of reactive hypoglycaemia.   There are probably more diabetic cookbooks around than there are for any diet controlled condition and they contain some very nutritious and imaginative recipes. In fact, they fulfil the nutritional requirements of those with POTS and MCAS.

Foods which are vasodilators and those which are vasoconstrictors

All foods have the ability to dilate or constrict blood vessels. Most of the time we don't think about the impact of nutrition on our blood pressure. Our autonomic nervous system seems to adjust quite well to a diversity of diets unless you have dysautonomia.

Most people are familiar with the knowledge that caffeine constricts blood vessels and, in doing so, it raises blood pressure. Caffeine is able to bind to adenosine receptors, for example, triggering blood vessels to constrict in the process.

Adenosine is a very powerful molecule that is related to sleep. It builds up throughout the day, attaching itself to adenosine receptors. As the day moves on, we get sleepier. When we drink a cup of caffeinated coffee, for example, it blocks off the receptors so that we remain alert.

Adenosine produces low blood pressure and late (probably reflex) tachycardia.

Reflex tachycardia is the phenomenon that occurs as blood pressure drops. The heart beats faster in an attempt to raise it and preserve oxygen supplies to the brain.

Decreases in blood volume through bleeding or dehydration would cause low blood pressure, too. If a mechanism for constricting blood vessels in order to raise blood pressure, is not available to the body, then tachycardia will occur.

Foods containing good amounts of adenosine are poultry, nuts and oily fish. Although these foods are clearly marketed as being 'good for you,' if you had a predisposition to POTS it may be that you need to include a wider variety of proteins that do not contain as much adenosine.

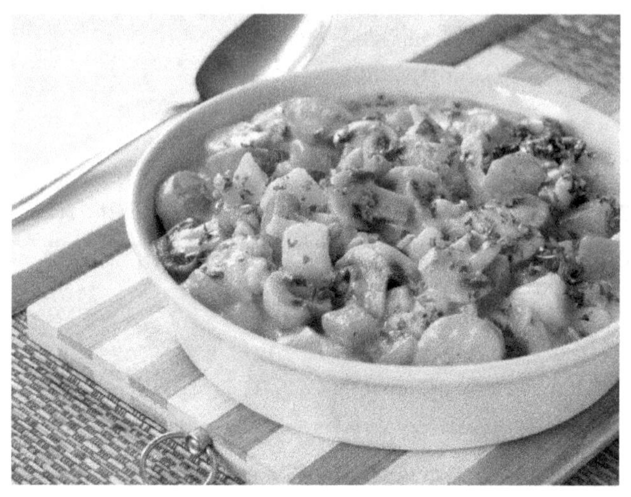

A dish containing chicken will contain good amounts of adenosine and may contribute to low blood pressure.

I used the knowledge that caffeine blocks adenosine receptors when I had a migraine. The dilated blood vessels were creating a fair amount of pain.

I had been quite miserable and fed up with the whole affair. I had an important meeting with my daughter in the town centre and sat in the café, waiting for her, feeling thoroughly dejected. A strong black cup of coffee came my way and I sipped it fitfully. Within ten minutes the pain had lifted and my smile returned. I could feel the migraine dissipating. It was nothing short of a miracle and a powerful lesson about the therapeutic effects of food.

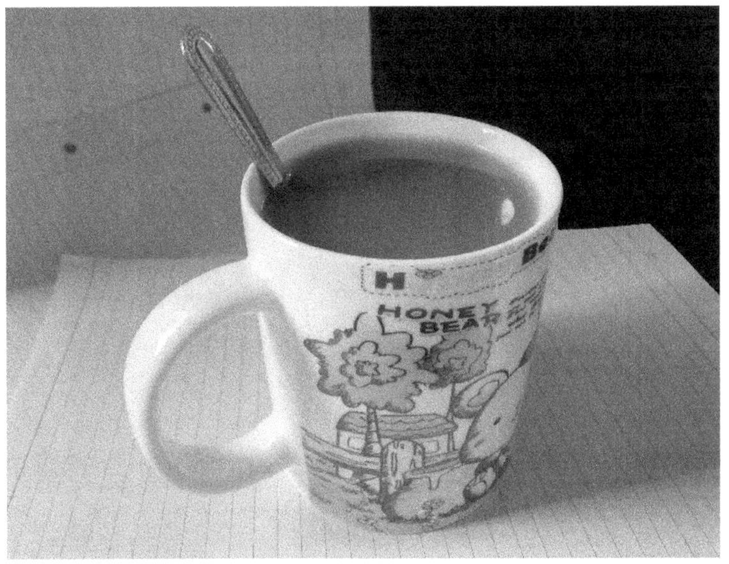

The caffeine in coffee will help to raise blood pressure and may prevent episodes of POTS.

It is quite likely that foods containing tyramine contribute to migraine and high blood pressure. Tyramine is a compound that results from the breakdown of the amino acid tyrosine.

When tyramine is present in the blood stream then the adrenal glands responds by sending chemical messengers into the bloodstream. These include the hormones, epinephrine and norepinephrine.

These hormones can dramatically elevate blood pressure and heart rate if foods containing tyrosine are eaten to excess in susceptible people.

They may have clear advantages for those with POTS. However, as a child, the very foods that can help increase blood pressure were also the ones that made me feel ill.

Tyrosine rich foods include:

- bananas
- fermented foods such as beer and wine
- figs
- prunes
- pineapples
- cheese – especially aged cheese
- raisins

In fact, any foods that are fermented, pickled, spoiled or aged.

These are considered vaso-constricting foods.

Many of the above foods not only contain tyramine but histamine too. As histamine is released from mast cells and may contribute to MACS, those with MACS associated POTS may not gain benefit from the above list of foods.

For such individuals we say that they are amine intolerant.

In contrast, there are other foods - besides foods containing adenosine - with a vaso-dilating effect. Many of them are high in magnesium which is a mineral that helps to widen blood vessels.

Magnesium deficiency is quite common in society. It is an important mineral involved in over 300 reactions in the body. It helps inhibit pain signals and this is useful knowledge because many NSAIDs such as ibuprofen activate mast cells. While they may afford some pain relief they could activate MCAS. Magnesium is a natural inhibitor of mast cell activation. Magnesium aids restful sleeps and dispels anxiety.

However, given magnesium's propensity to lower blood pressure it may not be the best treatment for those with a combination of POTS and MCAS.

The best sources of magnesium are nuts, beans and green leafy vegetables like chard and spinach.

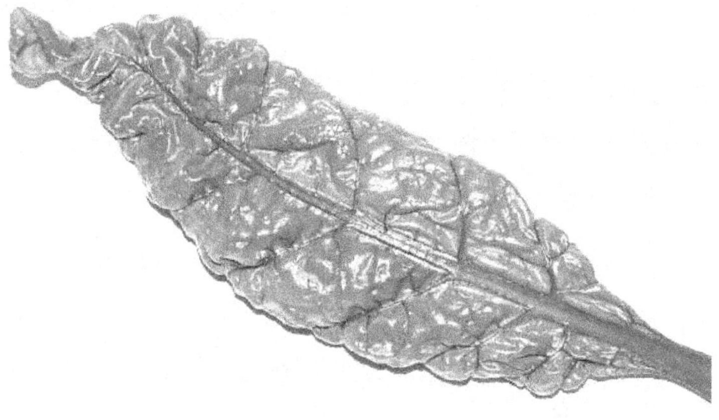

Chard is full of magnesium. People with POTS may have to limit their intake if it drops blood pressure too much.

Serotonin – a Jekyll and Hyde character

Serotonin is the hormone that most people refer to as the happy hormone. It is the hormone that pharmaceutical companies have targeted when producing the Selective Serotonin Reuptake Inhibitors (SSRI's) antidepressants. The most commonly heard of SSRI is Prozac.

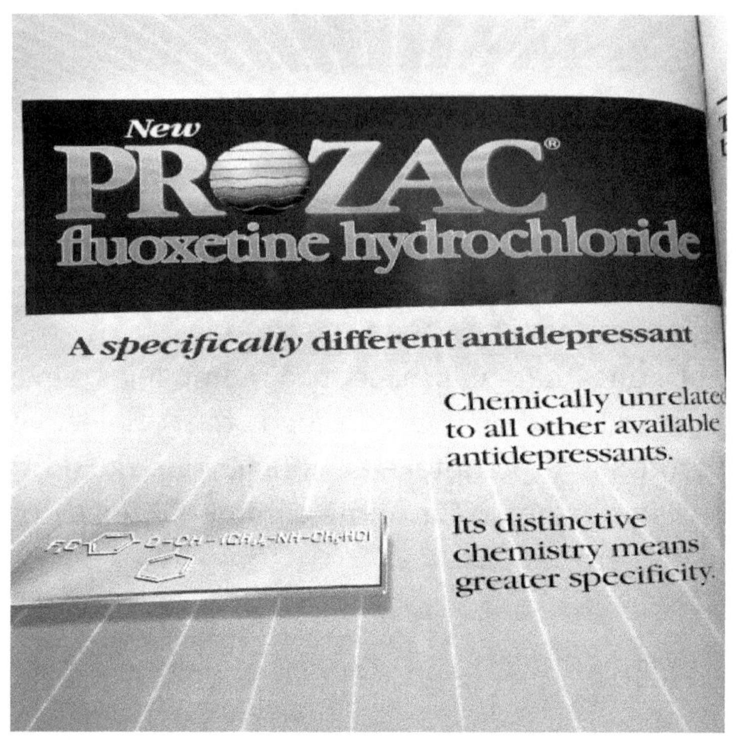

Serotonin's precursor is the amino acid tryptophan. Tryptophan has a number of different functions apart from being the parent amino acid of serotonin.

For example, tryptophan reduces anxiety and aids sleep.

However, in order for it to be converted to serotonin it requires iron, vitamin B2 and B6.

Serotonin in high concentrations acts as a vasoconstrictor and will raise blood pressure. It does this by potentiating the effects of other vasoconstrictors like norepinephrine.

A diet high in animal protein which contains tryptophan with the additional iron and B vitamins that are required may be all that it takes to keep the symptoms of POTS away.

In contrast, when serotonin is only available in much smaller amounts, it promotes the release of substances that act on smooth muscle to cause vasodilation. You can see this in action with fasting induced migraine. The supply of serotonin is reduced and in doing so dilates blood vessels which cause the intense pain of migraines.

 Thus a high carb diet (which contains less tryptophan) may help lower blood pressure and increase the likelihood of POTS at the same time.

Tryptophan does not cross the blood brain barrier easily and often does need to be accompanied by a little carbohydrate which helps to transport it across this barrier if we are to benefit from the anxiolytic and sleep inducing effects. This is why a glass of warm milk taken with a biscuit is recommended to aid sleep. The carbohydrate in the biscuit is the transporter for the tryptophan found in the milk

Tryptophan + iron/vitamins B2+ B6 = serotonin

Excess **SEROTONIN = HIGH BLOOD PRESSURE**

Limited serotonin = LOW BLOOD PRESSURE

Serotonin provides a fascinating insight into how food really is the only medicine that you need once you understand how to use that knowledge effectively. I believe that there should be more opportunities for students to learn about the amazing qualities of food. Here, in the UK, though, nutrition is no longer taught as part of the school curriculum.

Potassium also contributes to a lowering of blood pressure. It is a macro mineral, with electrolyte status, important for proper fluid balance, nerve transmission and muscle control.

The parameters of potassium requirements are quite narrow. Too low or too high potassium levels can have quite harmful effects.

For example, high potassium levels can cause:

- Muscle fatigue
- Arrhythmias
- Weakness

Which are not dissimilar to the symptoms of POTS.

Contributors to high potassium levels are:

- Dehydration (could be caused by potassium sparing diuretics) where potassium is concentrated in less fluid.
- Beta blockers
- Angiotensin receptor blockers
- Potassium supplements (I never recommend these)
- A diet very high in foods containing potassium if there is some underlying

abnormality such as kidney disease which causes a build- up of potassium
- Being heavy handed with salt substitutes such as Lo-salt which contain a combination of sodium chloride and potassium chloride.

Low potassium levels result in:

- Constipation
- Feeling of skipped heartbeat
- Paraesthesia (numbness and tingling)
- Palpitations
- Fatigue and weakness
- Muscle damage and spasms

I do not recommend using potassium supplements at any time for any reason. There is not a wide margin for its use and too much or too little potassium in the diet will quickly cause health problems such as cramping and weakness.

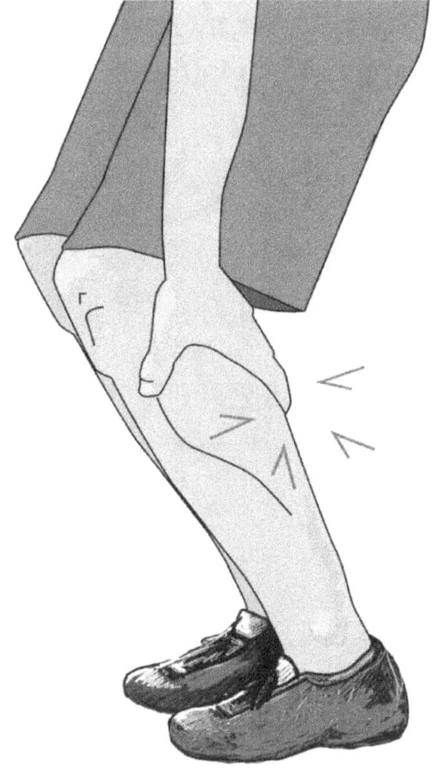

Low potassium levels can result in cramp and muscle spasms

Potassium is found in meat, milk, fresh fruit, whole grain and legumes.

We appear to have covered a lot of ground investigating foods that lower blood pressure or increase it and at this stage, I think it would be useful to tabulate it, with the mechanisms of action, so that the information is more accessible to you.

Table of foods or substances which particularly impact on blood pressure

Food/substance	Impact	Mechanism of

	on blood pressure	action
Magnesium Nuts and green leafy vegetables	Lowers blood pressure	Magnesium releases prostacyclin, a hormone like compound that reduces tension in the walls of blood vessels
Adenosine Poultry and nuts	Lowers blood pressure	There are many ways it can do this one of which is through inhibiting calcium entry into the cells through a specific type of calcium channel thus reducing calcium and causing

		relaxation of the blood vessel walls
Tyramine/tyrosine – aged, fermented, pickled and spoiled foods	Raises blood pressure	Tyramine targets adrenal glands which responds by increasing chemicals such as epinephrine which constrict blood vessels
caffeine	Raises blood pressure	Blocks adenosine receptors
serotonin	Both a blood pressure raising ((high serotonin levels) and blood pressure lowering	In high levels it helps increase the ability of norepinephrine to constrict blood vessel walls In lower

	action (low serotonin levels	quantities it acts on smooth muscle to cause vasodilation
Salted foods	Increases blood pressure	Salt attracts water and increases the volume of fluid that the heart must pump around the body
Potassium Fruit and vegetables, meat and bananas	Lowers blood pressure	Relaxes the blood pressure walls

Once you have studied POTS and MACS, it is fairly easy to see that there is a connection between them. It is a little harder – initially - to see a connection between them and the connective tissue disorder such as Ehlers Danlos Syndrome (EDS)

Nevertheless, such a connection is known to exist. In fact, there are a number of syndromes that appear to be connected to the syndromes of the subject matter of this book including irritable bowel syndrome and fibromyalgia syndrome. However, what is the connection between POTS and MACS and EDS?   That's the question we need to ask ourselves.

EDS, POTS and MCAS

Ehlers Danlos Syndrome is a heritable disease of connective tissue generally caused by mutations in connective tissue genes for collagen. Diet may play a part in the severity of the manifestation of this syndrome as environmental factors have greater influence on the outcome of genetic propensity than the rogue genes themselves.

Collagen is ubiquitous in the human body and one of its primary functions is to form part of the composition of the extracellular matrix which surrounds most cells.

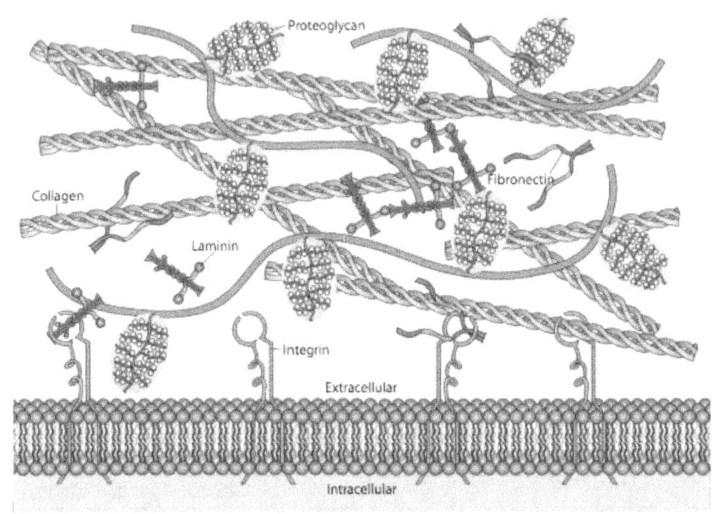

The extracellular matrix whose principle protein is collagen

The extra cellular matrix   provides structure as well as strength and elasticiy to the surrounding tissues. Hidden within it is a pathway known as the TGF – beta pathway which is important for the regulation and activation of the immune system. It is theorised that if the TGF-beta subunits are faulty then an inflammatory response could be triggered. Alternatively, if the structure of the extracellular matrix is compromised, any abnormalities may activate mast cells into releasing their contents.

This theory does provide some evidence for a connection with MCAS but it does not appear to be a particularly strong one. Nevertheless, mast cells do attach themselves to extra cellular matrix and poorly formed matrix may activate mast cells.

MCAS appears to be linked with EDS hypermobility type EDSh only. However, the TGF-beta anomaly can be found in other types so it is unclear whether the TGF-beta pathway anomaly is concerned with immune responses not connected to MCAS.

Although individuals with EDS do appear to have impaired immune systems studies have shown that the impairment appears to be connected with a deficiency of an immunoglobulin called IgG.

IgG is the main antibody which fights infection and **not** the antibody that is associated with allergies such as hay fever which is IgE.

Although allergic responses tend to be coordinated by IgE, there are some that do not involve IgE at all.

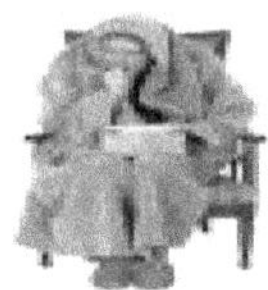

If you have a general infection caused by a virus or bacteria, then it would be IgG antibodies that would fight it.

Both types can be responsible for all the symptoms associated with allergies including itching, swelling and redness.

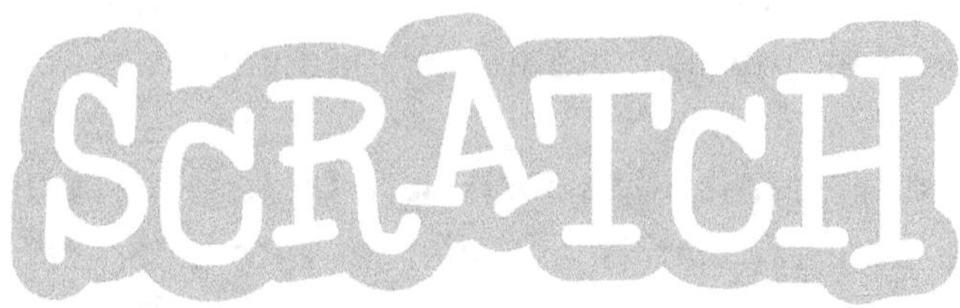

Reactions which involve IgE tend to involve protein fragments such as those found in peanut butter, cat dander and pollen.

Non IgE reactions which activate the release of the contents of mast cells could include heat and pressure. It may be an abnormality in tissue where over stretching activates sensitive mast cells. Reactions may occur due to abnormalities in the formation of a tissue.

If we accept that poor matrix formation can activate mast cells, then we would expect that MCAS would be present all the time. However, it is not. We may get episodes of it but then they tend to fade only to return later at some unspecified time.

From this, it is reasonable to assume that the structure of the extra cellular matrix is not permanently set in a particular form and has been influenced by external factors.

If we think about this, it applies to all tissues in our body. If we don't have enough calcium our bone structure will suffer. We may develop osteoporosis and in order to counteract this we may be prescribed vitamin D and calcium supplements.

Thus, what is a genetic leaning towards certain medical conditions does not necessarily manifest itself in certain environments. The greatest influences are those of environmental conditions.

 As a medical nutritionist I would also add that diet is a major environmental influencer in this regard as nutrients have the ability to turn genes on and off.

Mast cells are sensitive to cues. Even the over-stretching of a joint can cause the degranulation of their contents. However, if you can eat to strengthen and normalise the extracellular matrix which would reduce the sensitivity of mast cells to degranulate, then MACS simply could not occur if this was the particular activator of mast cells.

Of course, there may be many reasons why MACS occurs. Everyone will have their own specific triggers and we all have to adapt to our environments in order to minimise the impact of these on our lives.

Heat and pressure are particularly problematical for me. Sunlight causes angieoedema and urticaria and I adapt by avoiding too much sun and making air conditioning a priority for the house.

I know that if I go out walking my feet and lower legs will swell up. I might have to plan to take a larger pair of shoes with me or ones that can adapt to changing size.

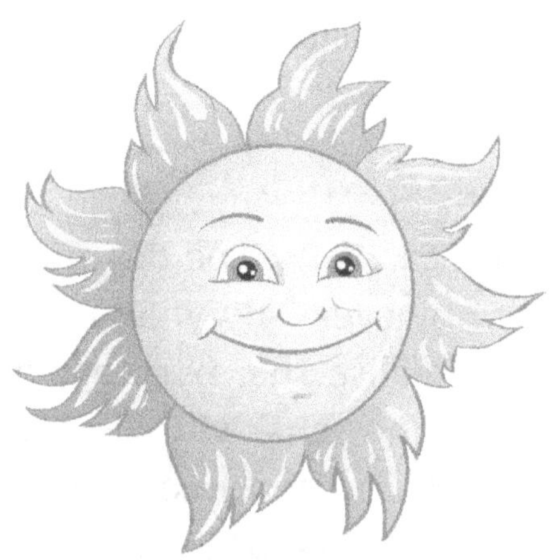

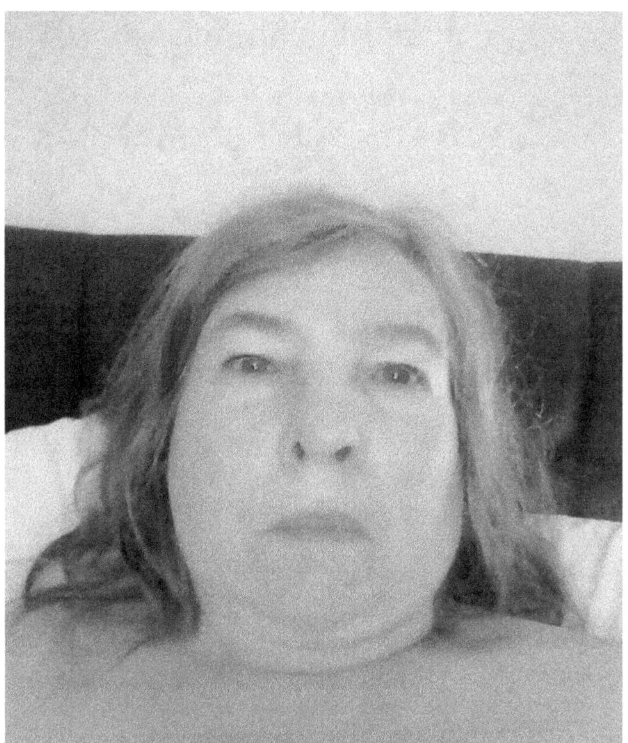

Facial flushing and sweating are characteristic of mast cell activation but this is not an IgE mediated response. There are non- IgE mediated responses and this has all the hallmarks of one.

The fragile tissues found in EDS which are so easily bruised or torn are perfect activators of mast cells.

A gentle knock which might go unnoticed by someone without a connective tissue disorder may result in extensive bruising in someone with EDS.

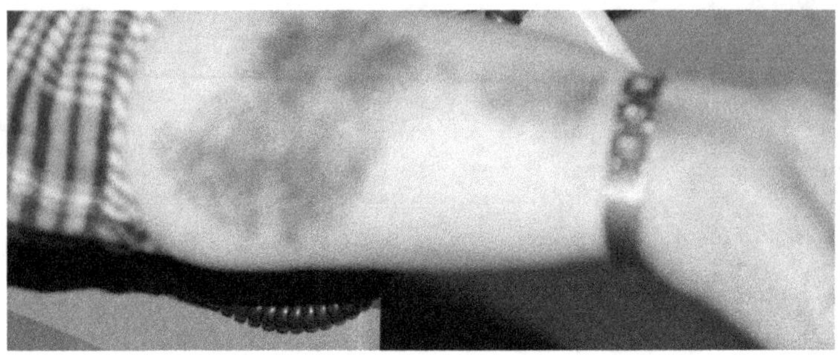

People with EDS do bruise easily – any slight knock has the potential to activate mast cells.

Although itchy eyes are often associated with an IgE related allergy. This isn't always the case.

Initially, my itchy eyes were put down to an allergy. I was prescribed sodium cromoglycate which is an excellent treatment for this type of thing. However, it didn't appear to work.

Following a consultation with my opthamologist and, as the sodium cromoglycate drops had not alleviated   my condition, I was prescribed carbomer gel given the amount of screen work that I did.

This gel was fine for three days doing much to alleviated the discomfort. I was pleased. I bought eight tubes but found the following day that I had developed a reaction to it (this probably **was** an IgE reaction).   My eye itched uncontrollably and streaked red every time I used it. I had to abandon it – and the other eight tubes much to my chagrin.

Now sodium cromoglycate, as my opthamologist will testify, is a remarkably good treatment for IgE mediated allergies. However, studies have shown that EDSers appear to have a propensity to non-IgE mediated allergies – in some cases, both - and, as such, different treatments may need to be prescribed. Therefore differentiating between the two forms of allergic responses is useful.

There is a fairly simple test that can decide whether a MCAS reaction is an IgE or a non IgE mediated reaction.

Typically, an IgE mediated reaction occurs within seconds or minutes of ingesting, or coming into contact with, the offending substance.

A non IgE mediated reaction is delayed and may take up to 48 hours to develop.

Both involve the immune system but the time frame in which they manifest themselves is very different.

In my case when I was eating anything, I felt the area around my neck tightening almost immediately. However, there were times when I would wake up flushed, sweating and with marked facial swelling long after I had eaten anything. That was caused by a non IgE reaction.

In both cases, avoidance of the offending trigger was essential but it was quercetin that actually transformed my life far better than the antihistamines and Tranexamic acid that I was prescribed.

Unfortunately, those with EDS are likely to show allergic type responses or side effects to medication which wouldn't bother people without a connective tissue disorder like EDS.

I found this out for myself after repeated trips to the immunology clinic to change prescribed medication that made me feel ill.

Initially, I had been prescribed Fenofexadine for angieodema. I suffered severe flu like symptoms on the three occasions that I took it. I can normally work through sickness, but this floored me. It impacted too much on my quality of life.

I returned to the clinic. I had been tested for 20 of the substances most likely to cause an allergic reaction but the results were not extraordinary.

Other antihistamines were also unacceptable in their side effects. I am a writer and researcher and did not take kindly to being in a permanently drug induced haze, the weight gain and the impact on bowel function.

I was also prescribed Tranexamic acid. This is a medication that assists the body's natural blood clotting process.

Even though it was designed for an entirely different purpose, Tranexamic acid appears to reduce the swelling that occurs in anaphylactic type reactions. Therefore, it is often prescribed for people with angieoedema. However, it has to be taken for a good number of months before the effects can be seen.

I did have mild swallowing problems which many with EDS do have. Tranexamic acid tablets can only be described as horse tablets. They come in only one size and there is not a liquid form of it either.

I found that I couldn't swallow them and spent one happy hour trying to get a tablet that was stuck to move further down my oesophagus. Water, milk and oil did not work. Repeated swallowing actions did not work. When I opened my mouth to try and tell my husband that he would have to take me to the hospital then it dislodged and I was able to swallow it properly.

 Tablets are coated for a purpose so that the contents will not touch delicate cells —and damage them - until they reach the stomach. They should never be broken and taken that way so I had to abandon these tablets because the manufacturers had not considered the impact on those with swallowing difficulties .

Tranexamic acid also had a number of side effects and these include:

- Pale skin

- trouble breathing with exertion

- unusual bleeding or bruising

- unusual tiredness or weakness

- change in vision

- chest pain or tightness

- confusion

- cough

- anxiety

- difficulty with swallowing

- lightheadedness

- fainting

- tachycardia

- numbness of the hands

- pain, redness, or swelling in the arm or leg

- puffiness or swelling of the eyelids or around the eyes, face, lips, or tongue

- urticaria itching

In fact, many of the symptoms that we are hoping to avoid in the first place.

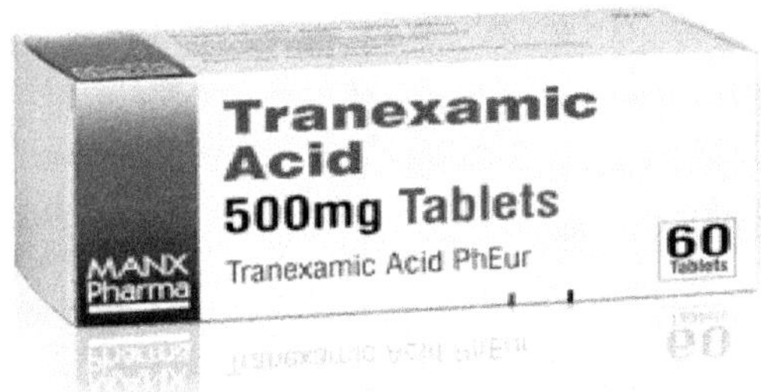

Tranexamic acid is sometimes used to treat angioedema

I did apologise profusely to the immunologist for this failing on my part although I secretly thought she should have known they would have been too difficult to swallow.

In the end I think the consultant immunologist felt just as traumatised as I did when I saw her.

On my last visit, I accepted the Certirizine and Epipen so that I could escape from the clinic. I think we had both had enough.

I put the medications   in my drawer. I went to the local store and bought quercetin. Good old quercetin. I have not had to use either Certirizine or Epipen since I started taking it.

Quercetin is unlikely to catch on, however – it would never make profits for the big pharmas.

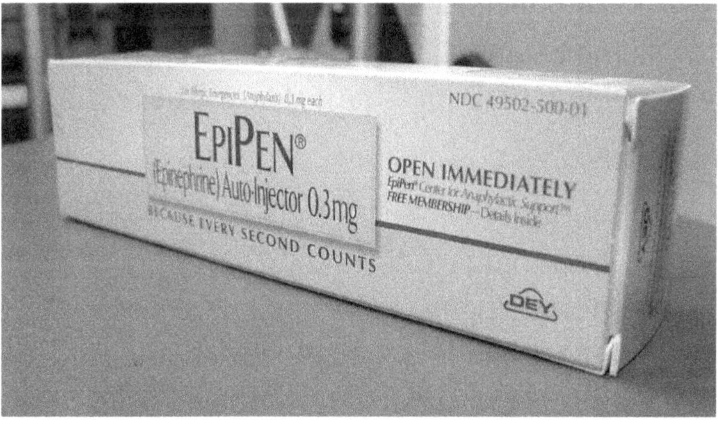

Epipens are prescribed for those who have life threatening anaphylaxis.

POTS and EDS

Many people with EDS experience POTS. It is a form of dysautonomia which is defined as a dysfunction of the autonomic nervous system.

The autonomic nervous system is responsible for all those bodily functions which occur without you thinking about them. These include:

- digestion
- breathing
- perspiring
- heart rate
- blood pressure
- sexual arousal
- dilation and constriction of blood vessels

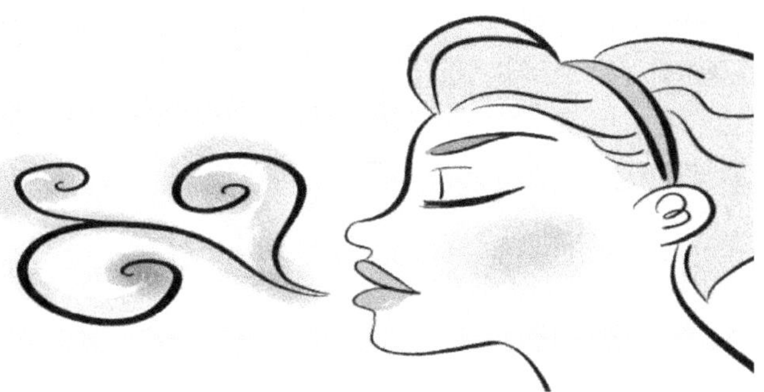

Breathing occurs as part of the autonomic nervous system's function

There are many theories why POTS occurs alongside EDS and I hope to cover some of them here.

It has been put forward that those with EDS become physically deconditioned due to to pain, frequent injury and fatigue. Tendonitis, for example, can keep people off their feet for extended periods of time and those with EDS tend to suffer from a lot of tendon damage.

When physically deconditioned the heart does not have the same leverage to increase the blood supply to the brain. However, as a well oxygenated supply of blood to the brain is vital, the heart rate increases so that the brain continues to be provided with enough oxygenated blood.

As women tend to suffer from POTS more than men and have smaller hearts which would decondition more quickly, then the above theory has some merit.

There are slightly double the figures of women with EDS to men in the ratio of 70:30 so this supports the theory although differences in hormones may also account for the above.

Vitamin B12 deficiency is often found in those with EDS as well as POTS sufferers. Studies on adolescent groups have found that low vitamin B12 levels are associated with POTS.

A deficiency of this vital nutrient can lead to sympathetic nervous system baroreceptor dysfunction. Baroreceptors are, of course, responsive to pressure and when they dysfunction they cannot regulate the normal chemical pathways involving epinephrine.

Epinephrine, as we have already learned, constricts blood vessel walls increasing blood pressure as it does so.

A lack of vitamin B12 leaves the sympathetic nervous system unable to respond to postural changes.

As people age they are unable to absorb vitamin B12 as well as they could do when younger. Vitamin B12 needs to be separated from its protein source, once it is eaten, but this requires an acidic environment in which to happen.

Stomach acid becomes less acidic as you age and you also produce less of it.

 Lax sphincter muscles mean that some acid reflux may occur so that the sufferer reaches for the proton pump inhibitors or the antacids which normally contain calcium or magnesium in order to curb their indigestion.

These factors all contribute to an environment where B!2 cannot be separated from its protein source to be used.

As we have already seen though, adolescents and POTS appear to be associated. Why do adolescents appear to be susceptible to POTS?

The adolescent years are a time when parental guidance has less influence. Teenagers are keen to use their new found freedom to explore aspects of culture that they hadn't had the freedom to do before.

Vegetarianism or veganism has become popular. It has fuelled by news that there will soon not be enough meat to feed the planet. Teenagers want to do their bit and can be enthusiastic in doing so. However, sometimes enthusiasm overshadows the need to do a little research on what particular problems may occur if meat is left out of the diet.

Vitamin B12 is a nutrient that can only be obtained from animal sources.

Vitamin D is only obtainable from very few sources and only one plant source – irradiated mushrooms.

Zinc, a marvellous trace mineral involved in the synthesis of over one thousand enzymes or macromolecules binds to phytates – a naturally occuring substance in all plants and cannot be used by the body.

Any diet which excludes certain food groups needs to be thoroughly investigated to ascertain whether sound nutrition is possible and how this will be incorporated into the diet. When you consider that zinc is responsible for the synthesis of well over a thousand enzymes and macromolecules a deficiency will be life changing for all the wrong reasons.

Many teenagers I have met who are ardent supporters of vegetarianism or veganism are also iron deficient.

Vitamin B12 injections are often the easiest and most reliable way to correct a deficiency. There are also lozenges which can be placed between gum and upper lip so that the vitamin can be absorbed directly into the blood stream that way.

As vitamin B12 deficiency is quite common, then anyone with a history of syncope or chronic fatigue should automatically be screened for this.

There is also an autoimmune disease called pernicious anaemia which creates a vitamin B12 deficiency. Prior to the advent of vitamin B12 injections, sufferers had to eat a couple of pounds of raw liver daily. Without this source of vitamin B12 they would have died.

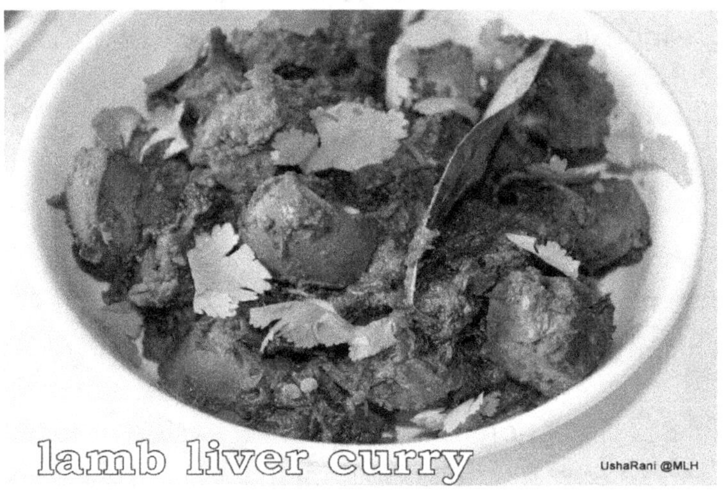

Lamb's liver is a delight and full of vitamin B12

While we are on the subject of B vitamins we need to take a look at another one – that of vitamin B6 - which is involved in the synthesis of the extracellular matrix. As such a pyroxidine (B6) deficiency may provide a connection between the puzzling syndromes we are currently investigating .

A study was carried out on fast growing male chicks to see if vitamin B6 deprivation affected the extra cellular matrix

. At six weeks the chicks were deprived of pyroxidine in their feed, but not to the point where neurological symptoms were evident.

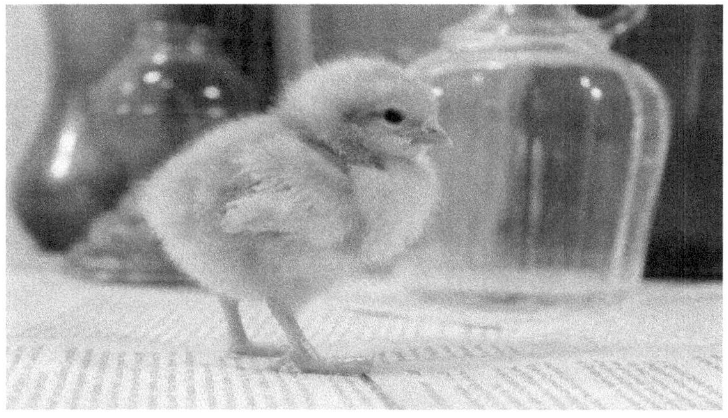

When the extracellular matrix was examined under a light microscope, it showed abnormalities in the connective tissue. This would not be surprising since vitamin B6 is essential for collagen synthesis. Pyroxidine deficiency results in low amounts of aldehydes and these are necessary for cross link formation in the matrix.

If a pyroxidine deficiency can result in abnormal matrix this abnormality may be enough to cause mast cells to activate and release their contents. It provides a plausible reason for th connection between hypermobile EDS and MCAS.

Normally, if there is a known deficiency of one of the B vitamins then others are likely to occur since the different B vitamins tend to work synergistically and can generally be found in the same foods

Good sources of vitamin B6 and vitamin B12 can be found in the lists below.

List of foods containg vitamins B6 or B12

Good sources of vitamin B6	Good sources of vitamin B12
<ul><li>turkey</li><li>pork</li><li>halibut</li><li>sirloin steak</li><li>chicken</li><li>salmon</li><li>banana</li><li>liver is a good source of the B vitamins</li></ul>	<ul><li>meat especially lightly cooked liver</li><li>fish</li><li>mile</li><li>eggs</li><li>cheese</li><li>fortified breakfast cereals</li></ul>

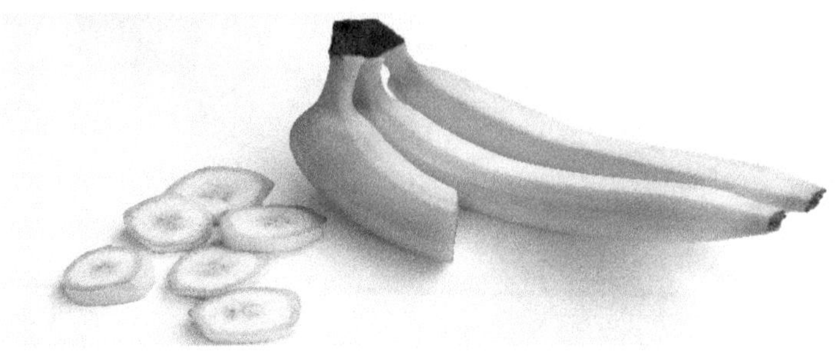

Bananas contain vitamin B6

We have seen the importance of eating a well balanced diet but is it that easy to include all nutrients in optimum amounts or is it possible that some nutrients may be much harder to obtain than others.

For our final look at the connection between our three syndromes we are going to look at vitamin D. At one time vitamin D deficiency was unlikely but this was the time when we did not commute to work in cars or stay cooped up in offices so that we did not benefit from the sunlight and the free vitamin D it produced.

If there is ever an example of how environmental factors can impact our health then vitamin D is it.

People are well aware that vitamin D has something to do with healthy bones and teeth. They may even know that if you have a chest infection then cod liver oil can be helpful as it abounds in vitamins A and D. Beyond that, there are very few who know that there is published data on vitamin D which provides evidence that vitamin D deficiency could cause the development of POTS.

In order to understand how this works you will need a little understanding of catecholamines.

Catecholamines are simply various type of hormone which are made in the adrenal glands. The adrenal glands are situated above the kidneys.

The most well known catecholamines are:

- dopamine
- norepinephrine
- adrenalin

When you are physically or emotionally stressed the adrenal glands send appropriate catecholamines into the blood stream.

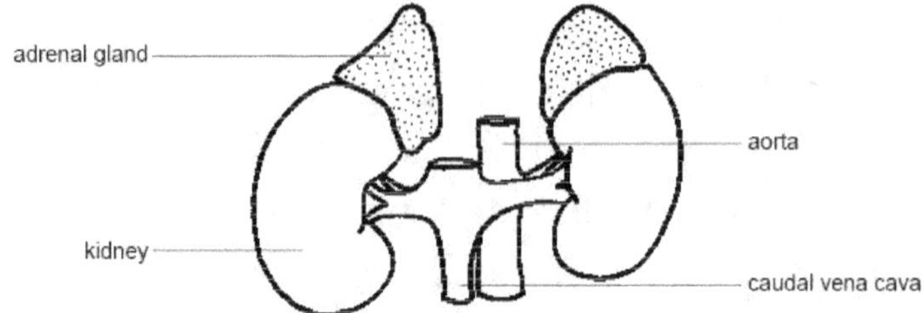

A deficiency of vitamin D causes an alteration in catecholamine levels via activity in the sympathetic nervous system. An imbalance of norepinephrine and adrenalin occurs with lower levels of the latter.

The lower levels of adrenalin mean that vasoconstriction – with subsequent raised blood pressure – cannot respond properly to the changing positions which bring about episodes of POTS.

However, it is vital that the brain is oxygenated. The only option left to prevent any neurological damage is for the heart rate to increase.

Thus there is a tachycardic - as opposed to a hypertensive - response based on the amount of available vitamin D.

Vitamin D deficiency = tachycardia

Vitamin D sufficiency = hypertensive response

Now, I have mentioned previously that vitamin D is found in very few foods such as:

- egg yolks

- liver

- irradiated mushrooms

- oily fish

However, you would have to eat quite large amounts, on a daily basis, in order to get the recommended daily allowance.

Most of our vitamin D is obtained through the action of the sun's rays on our skin. Our enthusiasm for slip slap slopping sun tan lotion all over us hinders our ability to make vitamin D.

There are so many hindrances to us making vitamin D or absorbing it in our diet.

- elderly people do not absorb any nutrient optimally. This is part of the ageing process so food has to be nutrient dense They tend to eat less. They do not synthesise vitamin D from the sun's rays as well as they did when they were younger.

- Individuals with darker skin tend to absorb less of the sun's rays. The melanin is there to protect skin from sun damage but it also inhibits the synthesis of vitamin D

- People with absorption problems such as Crohn's disease or cystic fibrosis are also at risk of vitamin D deficiency

- As fat in the diet is required to absorb vitamin D, then those on low fat diets are also susceptible.

There are two forms of vitamin D. The non-active form 25(OH)D is mainly converted to the active form D3 in the kidney. However, it is recognised that conversion of inactive to active vitamin D does occur in other tissues to a lesser extent.

A vitamin D deficiency can also increase the risk of MCAS. Optimum amounts of vitamin D increase the receptors found on the surface of mast cells. This aids stabilisation of mast cells. Without sufficient vitamin D to provide stability, mast cells become decidedly twitchy and are activated by the slightest little thing.

By now, it may not surprise you that the active form of vitamin D also impacts collagen synthesis. It undertakes this by stimulating the expression of this protein. Thus, a deficiency of D3 may well contribute to the poor formation of connective tissue which is not just confined to bones and joints we normally associate it with.

The manifestation of EDS, MCAS and POTS could all be explained by a lack of vitamin D and it is such an easy nutrient to suffer a deficiency from.

When we look at the impact of environmental factors, they include:

- Mainly working indoors

- Low fat diets

- The lack of inclusion of liver in the diet when it was very much a part of diets during the world wars.

- Low fat diets because of the mistaken belief that saturated fat is bad for us.

- Replacing lard (which contains vitamin D) with inflammation causing omega 6 vegetable oils.

- Less pie making (using lard) because it is erroneously believed that pastry made with lard is bad for us.

- Using sun tan lotion

This list is by no means a definitive list but it illustrates how much what we experience health wise is as a result of environmental factors more than what is written in our genes.

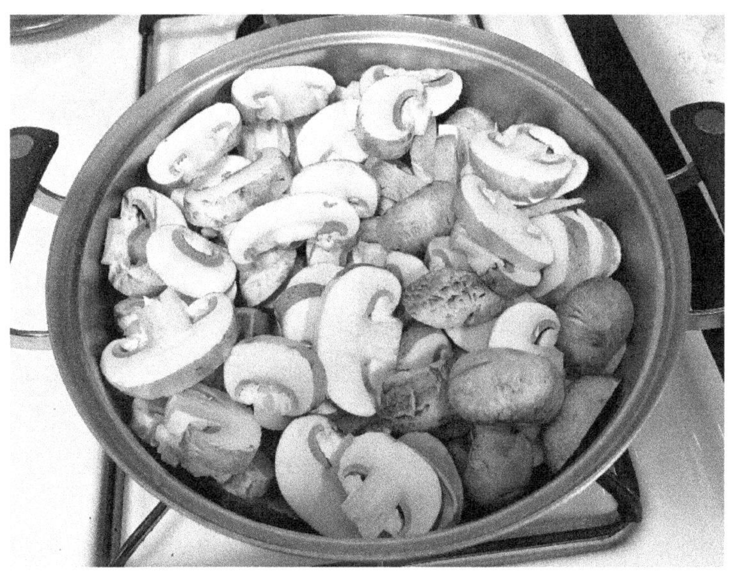

Irradiated mushrooms are full of vitamin D

Although all the associations connecting EDS, POTS and MCAS cannot be made in a book of this size, the enduring theme is that nutrition makes a huge impact on health. In addition, I have included the potential causative factors which are more common and easier to address.

Correct nutrition can make a condition that has relapsed, go into remission. There it may stay for the rest of your life if you continue to address the deficiencies that caused the diseases manifestation in the first place.

We are more well acquainted with the idea of relapses and remissions in multiple sclerosis but these aberrations happen in many chronic diseases. We may refer to them as 'flare ups' but they do not happen out of the blue. There is a reason for them and the reasons need to be explored and addressed.

Individuals with an investigative personality will probably enjoy this type of thing. I have always had an inquisitive mind constantly wanting to know what would happen if I did this or that. It has worked well for me and I adapted my diet and lifestyle over a period of months so that I did not have to rely on prescription medicines.

When I look back at my younger self with so many painful symptoms of EDS, multiple allergies, angieoedema and a tendency to syncope - often at the most inconvenient times - I hardly recognise myself because that person barely exists now.

I have included four daily supplements in my daily regime. These are:

- Vitamin D – 2000 iu's daily
- Magnesium 400mg daily
- Quercetin 500mg daily
- Zinc 12 -25mg daily

I eat a leafy green vegetable every day and use saturated fats instead of omega 6 vegetable oils.

Apart from that, very little has changed apart from I no longer suffer from repeated bouts of EDS related tendonitis which, for me, was the most debilitating symptom out of many that I had.

I no longer have MCAS or POTS, either which has meant that I am less restricted when I am going out.

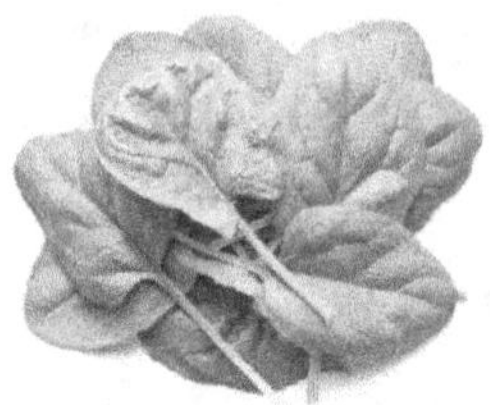

It's a good habit to eat a leafy green vegetable every day.

Many of my family members, going back many generations have EDS, MCAS and POTS with varying degrees of severity. In that respect we know that there is a heritable aspect to it but the good news is that we are not ultimately defined by our genetic inheritance. It is up to us to investigate and find the key to our own unique set of problems and adapt our environment accordingly.

Thiamine Deficiency: the great mimicker

This book cannot end without looking at the impact of thiamine, the great mimicker of….. well everything. A deficiency can be associated with apparently unrelated symptoms. It impacts every single cell in your body so what is thiamine and how does it function?

Thiamine is the first of the B vitamins to be identified and is therefore known as B1. It is vital for energy synthesis in the mitochondria where it provides the spark plug to ignite oxygen and energy in these organelles.

Thiamine deficiency is associated with beriberi of which there are three that are well-recognised. There is dry beriberi where there is central nervous involvement, wet beriberi where the thiamine deficiency has definitely impacted the cardiovascular system and gastrointestinal beriberi which can impact any part of the gastrointestinal system.

Thiamine causes acid producing cells in the stomach to release that acid. The stomach needs to be acidic for many reasons including:

Vitamin B12 cannot be separated from its protein souce without being in an acidic environment

An acidic environment is required to close the valve at the top of the stomach without which stomach acid would leak causing heartburn or indigestion.

An acidic environment is needed to open the valve at the bottom of the stomach to allow digested contents to pass into the small intestine. Without this valve allowing the contents to pass through, partially digested food would sit in the stomach causing bloating and abdominal distension.

Without sufficient thiamine then the vagus nerve cannot work properly so that the digestive responses which are normally rhythmic and effective, become sluggish and uncoordinated causing abdominal discomfort and intractable constipation.

I have known people be on three or four bowel medications and, in one case, have to use an anal irrigation system before being placed on thiamine. Two weeks later they report bowel sounds and around the 7 weeks or 2 months mark their bowel movements had returned to normal. Now that truly is a miracle.

So having learned a little of the impact of thiamine on the gastrointestinal system we can now look at how thiamine is involved in MCAS. Thiamine isn't so straightforward. Some people benefit greatly from it and others finds it worsens their symptoms. However, given thiamine's benefits in enabling sleep through its production of gamma amino butyric acid and providing pain relief, it is worth trying.

Other people have reported better balance with one 75 year old who could only walk up and down steps holding onto a rail, finding that he could skip up and down the steps within two weeks of starting high dose thiamine.

Another lady wrote:

I hope you don't mine me messaging you. I have to get this out there. Your advice on the thiamine and magnesium supplements has brought about the best result for me. For 3 years I have suffered numbness and pins and needles in my feet. First diagnosed as Morton's Neuroma. Then sciatica. Then neuropathy. Amitryptyline prescribed. Yes, I can sleep but groggy and no improvement. 2 weeks on B1 and magnesium and I'm almost symptom free.   I walk much better, more flexible a transformation. Thank you a million times over.

Charlotte writes:

I know that I'm only on my third day of taking 500mg of thiamin but I have only taken half the amount of my gabapentin and only half the amount of tramadol – I sure hope that I get to the point I don't need my prescribed meds!!!

So the benefits are there but some people do state that they did not derive any benefit from thiamine. Some even said it worsened their condition.

The reason that thiamine did not appear to work is because it has not been taken with an activator. In thiamine's case it is magnesium and without sufficient magnesium in the diet then thiamine is not activated and is therefore useless.

Every substance in the body depends on many other trace elements and vitamins in order to be able to function.

In addition, there are foods and beverages which degrade thiamine so that it cannot work. These include:

Alcohol

Tea and coffee

Raw fish (sushi and shellfish)

High carbohydrate diets.

Jean wrote:

I didn't know about the food and drink that degrades thiamine. I liked drinking coffee. First thing I did when I got up in the morning, two cups of strong black coffee, a glass or wine or two on the evening. I've always enjoyed shellfish too. When I reduced all these and took them away from the time that I took the thiamine and magnesium, I felt the effect almost immediately. I had the best night's sleep I had for a long time.   The MCAS disappeared totally since. I didn't quite believe it so I stopped the thiamine and the MCAS came back. I'm going to make sure that I keep my thiamine levels topped up now. I no longer suffer from PoTS either.

Thiamine is found in:

Dried brewer's yeast

Yeast extract

Brown rice

Pork muscle meat

Nuts – especially pistachios

Oats

Liver especially pork liver

Wholemeal bread (although the carbohydrate content of flour may reduce the amount available to the body.

Thiamine is quite a vulnerable vitamin and is easily lost through cooking and heat.

The effect of thiamine has been said to be similar to that of Modafinil which is used by students to aid learning and prevent mental fatigue.

Thiamine can be injected or supplemented as it's quite difficult to take in enough to correct a

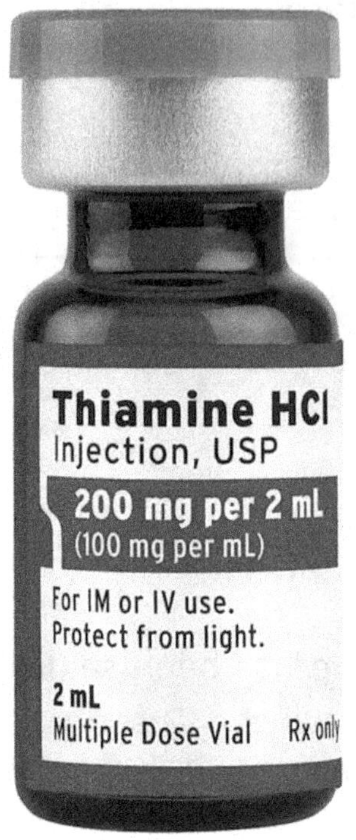

Deficiency. Once a deficiency has been corrected then it is fine to reduce thiamine until you are able to manage by increasing foods which contain good amounts of thiamine as well as remembering not to have too many which degrade thiamine. High carbohydrate diets are a problem in society at the moment. It is better to veer towards a keto diet which consists mainly of animal protein, fat and a small amount of low carbohydrate veg – generally green leafy vegetables.

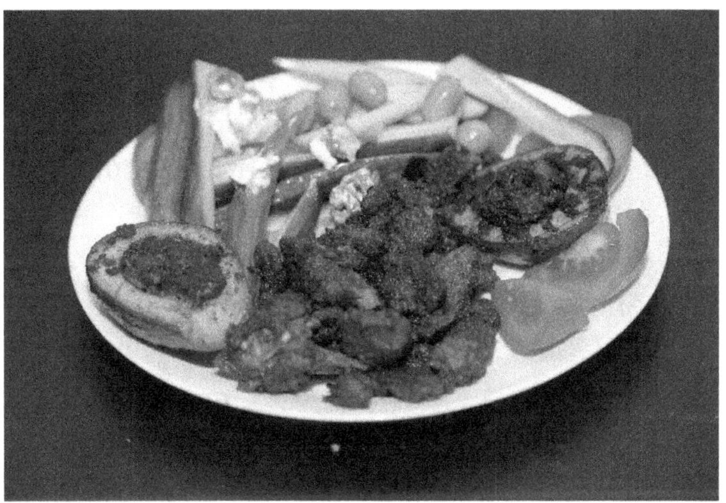

A typical keto meal.

Thiamine has superior pain relieving properties and helps GABA production which has significant analgesic and calming effects as well as aiding sleep.

There are analogues of GABA in the form of the medications gabapentin and pregabalin but these do not appear to cross the blood brain barrier and can cause rapid weight gain which does not happen with thiamine.

Thiamine really can help address the pain that those with EDS live with on a day to day basis with some describing thiamine as 'melting away the pain.

Thiamine deficiency is also associated with the tachycardia which those with PoTS often complain of. A few days of thiamine brings welcome relief. Wet beriberi is the cardiovascular form of thiamine deficiency and symptoms often match some of those found in the conditions that are the subject of this book. They include:

Increased heart rate

Swelling of the lower legs

Shortness of breath during activity

Awakening at night with shortness of breath

Dry beriberi which is related to the nervous system has symptoms which include:

Difficulty walking

Vomiting

Tingling

Nystagmus

Pain

Mental confusion and brain fog

Speech difficulties[1]

Poor muscle function which may progress to paralysis of the lower legs.

I think many readers of this book will recognise some of these symptoms. In addition, there is enough research that confirms that a group of individuals with PoTs do have a thiamine deficiency.

The thiamine regime which works so well consists of:

Thiamine 300mg

---

[1] https://faseb.onlinelibrary.wiley.com/doi/abs/10.1096/fasebj.2019.33.1_supplement.871.3

Magnesium 300mg

A good B complex

The thiamine can be taken in divided doses and after a month or two the dose can be reduced to 100mg daily. Most supplements come in 100mg.

As you will have concluded the symptoms which accompany EDS do not necessarily have the same underlying cause. However, nutrients are a major environmental factor which can change the course - and severity – of a condition. Nutrients impact the epigenome and can turn on or off a genetic propensity to a condition, Often the 'relapses' of symptoms are nothing more than a particular nutrient which has been eaten in lesser quantities for some meals but which is needed to keep the symptoms at bay.

It's helpful to keep a diary and look for patterns which worsen or improve your condition. No two persons are the same and what works for one may not work for another. It's a challenge but one, I think, that is worth it in order to live life in the fullest that it can be.

Other books by this author include:

- The EDS and Hypermobility Syndrome Diet
- Alleviating Symptoms of EDS
- Gastroparesis
- The EDS recipe book

- The Lipoedema Diet
- The Lymphoedema Diet: reverse and repair lymphatic damage
- The Anti Virus Diet
- The Asthma Diet
- The Reluctant Bowel
- The MND Diet
- The Alzheimer's and Vascular Dementia Disease Diet
- Why we live longer with higher cholesterol levels
- The Metabolic Syndrome Diet
- Parkinson's Disease: dietary changes that work
- https://www.amazon.co.uk/dp/B07TBHMV6N

Among many others

They are available on Amazon

Lynne has written a semi-autobiographical trilogy.

While this trilogy is available on kindle and paperback on Amazon, it may be cheaper to buy from the link below.

They may be obtained off the publisher's website, in paperback form, where they are more reasonably priced.

https://www.shieldcrest.co.uk/?s=lynne+d+m+noble++

For the full range of books by this author, visit the author website on

https://www.amazon.co.uk/-/e/B07BPQZ5CD

https://www.amazon.com/-/e/B07BPQZ5CD

The Exodus Project

My first introduction to the far reaching impact of The Exodus Project occurred when I was travelling around Cawthorne in one of their buses, visiting gardens. A young lad was happily munching on a sandwich. He looked up briefly, pointed to the driver and said,' He's my second dad, he is,' then he returned to his sandwich without further comment

Such remarks are often very telling and so I arranged to meet Jackie Peel and Martin Sawdon, at the charity's premises in Barnsley. They set up the Exodus Project 20 years ago. They moved into their current premises – a redundant Methodist church - in 2010.

Both Jackie and Martin have been youth workers in their church. Martin worked in housing for the homeless in addition to working in learning disabilities services in institutional settings.

The work that the Exodus Project undertakes is of paramount importance to the communities it serves. These were former mining communities which became disadvantaged after pit-closures. Currently about 400 children attend mid-week activities from Monday to Thursday inclusive. These activities include dance, drama, craft, music, sports and games. In addition, there are weekend camps, cycle treks, outward bound activities, bowling and swimming. The children are taught valuable life skills including how to cook and bake. It is all about teaching children how to fulfil their potential and learn skills they will be able to pass onto the next generation.

The grounds, once overgrown, have been turned into a play- and camping - ground. A miniature railway is in the process of being installed.

Martin and Jackie have developed a unique model in that The Exodus Project goes beyond dispensing services. They are keen to build up relationships with the whole family and not just the child that attends the mid- week clubs. In addition, once children have reached the age of fourteen, they are invited to help out with the younger groups as junior volunteers. Once they reach the age of eighteen, they become adult volunteers. This model provides a constant supply of help from individuals who have benefitted already from attending such groups.

The building is large and inviting. It is decorated with bold colours and has comfy seating. It is a real home from home; a haven for families who have been disadvantaged by the closure of the life force of its community.

Martin and Jackie have clear ideas about how they wish to develop the Exodus Project but the lottery funding which they benefitted from is no longer available. Sadly, they have had to close two of their clubs due to lack of funding. This decision wasn't taken lightly. They do have two charity shops which raises some money and they obtain some funding from outside organisations for the use of their facilities. However, this is clearly not enough to keep their clubs, weekend activities and building going to cater for the ever growing number of children who are benefitting from the work being undertaken here.   Neither does it allow for future development.

Exodus do have a Just Giving page which can be found here if you wish to help further their work https://www.justgiving.com/exodus

In addition, you can keep up with activities on their Facebook page here

https://www.facebook.com/search/top/?q=the%20exodus%20project%20barnsley&epa=SEARCH_BOX

Lynne's blog and twitter posts can be found here:

https://quintessentiallylynne.weebly.com/nutritional-medicine.html

twitter: Lynne D M Noble@ldmn53